CONTENTS

Copyright 1
Introduction 1
Chapter 1: Why Women's Health Matters 1
Chapter 2: Hormonal Health..1
Chapter 3: Reproductive Health 1
Chapter 4: Women's Sexual Health 1
Chapter 5: Mental Health and Well-being for Women 1
Chapter 6: Physical Fitness and Well-being for Women 1
Chapter 7: Nutrition and Healthy Eating Habits for Women 1
Chapter 8: Self-Care and Stress Management for Women...................1
Chapter 9: Women's Empowerment and Self-Confidence 1
Chapter 10: Maintaining Healthy Relationships and Fostering a
Supportive Community of Women..1
Chapter 11: Integrative and Complementary Therapies.....................1
Chapter 12. Empowerment and Self-Advocacy 1
Conclusion...1
The Women's Health Code 1

THE WOMEN'S HEALTH CODE

Unveiling the Untold Realities of Women's Wellness

Dr. Laura Campbell

COPYRIGHT

INTRODUCTION

Welcome to "The Women's Health Code: Unveiling the Untold Realities of Women's Wellness" This book is a journey into the vast landscape of women's health, designed to equip you with valuable knowledge, practical strategies, and empowering insights to enhance your physical, mental, and emotional well-being. In these pages, we will explore the unique health needs of women, addressing the various stages and aspects of a woman's life, and providing guidance for achieving a balanced and fulfilling lifestyle.

CHAPTER 1: WHY WOMEN'S HEALTH MATTERS

Women's health is a vital and complex subject, encompassing a range of physical, mental, and emotional aspects specific to women's biology and life experiences. It is crucial to recognize that women have distinct health needs and considerations that differ from those of men. By understanding and addressing these unique aspects, we can optimize our health, prevent illnesses, and promote overall well-being.

Throughout history, women's health has often been underrepresented or overlooked, and women themselves have faced various challenges in obtaining appropriate care and support. This book seeks to bridge that gap by empowering women with knowledge and resources to take control of their health and make informed decisions.

Understanding the Unique Health Needs of Women

Women experience remarkable physiological changes throughout their lives, from puberty to pregnancy, menopause, and beyond. These changes bring with them specific health concerns and considerations that deserve attention and proactive management.

One of the key areas we will delve into is hormonal health. The intricate dance of hormones in a woman's body influences her menstrual cycle, fertility, and overall well-being. We will explore the phases of the menstrual cycle, common hormonal imbalances, and natural approaches to balancing hormones, empowering you to better understand and support your body's hormonal fluctuations.

Reproductive health is another crucial aspect we will explore in this book. From family planning and fertility awareness to preconception care and pregnancy, we will delve into the various factors that contribute to reproductive health and provide practical advice for optimizing fertility, maintaining a healthy pregnancy, and nurturing the mother-child bond.

The journey of a woman continues beyond reproductive years, leading to menopause and its accompanying changes. We will navigate the transitions and challenges of perimenopause and menopause, discussing symptom management, hormonal changes, and strategies for maintaining overall well-being during this transformative stage of life.

Mental and emotional well-being is an integral part of women's health. Women are more prone to stress, anxiety, and mood disorders due to various factors such as hormonal fluctuations, societal pressures, and life circumstances. We will explore strategies to address stress, manage anxiety, and cultivate emotional resilience and self-care practices that promote mental well-being.

Women's sexual health is another vital aspect that deserves attention and open discussion. Understanding female sexual anatomy and function, addressing common sexual health concerns, and enhancing intimacy and sexual well-being are important for nurturing healthy relationships and embracing one's sexuality with confidence and satisfaction.

Proper nutrition and eating habits play a significant role in women's health. We will discuss balanced eating for optimal energy and vitality, highlight key nutrients crucial for women's health, and explore approaches to managing weight and promoting healthy body image, fostering a positive relationship with food and nourishing your body.

Physical fitness and exercise are integral components of a healthy lifestyle. We will guide you in customizing a fitness routine tailored to women's needs, emphasizing the benefits of strength training, cardiovascular exercise, and physical activity for women's health.

Whether you are a beginner or an experienced fitness enthusiast, this book will provide insights to support your journey toward a stronger, more active life.

Preventive care and screenings are essential for early detection and management of potential health issues. We will discuss the importance of regular check-ups, preventive measures for common women's health concerns, and the significance of cancer prevention and early detection.

As women, we face specific health challenges such as breast health, osteoporosis, and heart disease. Navigating these concerns requires knowledge and proactive measures. We will explore strategies for maintaining breast health, optimizing bone health, and understanding heart health to empower you in safeguarding your well-being.

In addition to conventional approaches, we will also delve into integrative and complementary therapies. Exploring alternative and holistic approaches, herbal remedies, and integrating mind-body practices into healthcare will provide you with a well-rounded understanding of the possibilities for supporting your health and well-being.

Lastly, this book emphasizes the importance of empowerment and self-advocacy. Taking charge of your health, building a supportive healthcare team, and accessing resources for women's health and support are integral to your journey toward optimal well-being.

By delving into these topics and empowering yourself with knowledge, you are taking a significant step toward becoming an informed and active participant in your own health and well-being. Let this book serve as a guide, a resource, and a source of inspiration as you embark on this transformative journey toward a healthier, happier, and more empowered you.

Now, let's begin our exploration of women's health, empowering ourselves with the knowledge and tools to lead vibrant and fulfilling lives.

Remember, you have the power to shape your health destiny. Let's embark on this journey together!

CHAPTER 2: HORMONAL HEALTH

The intricate dance of hormones within a woman's body influences numerous aspects of her health and well-being. From regulating the menstrual cycle to influencing fertility, mood, energy levels, and more, hormones play a vital role in women's lives. In this chapter, we will explore the phases of the menstrual cycle, common hormonal imbalances in women, and natural approaches to balancing hormones.

The Menstrual Cycle and Its Phases

The menstrual cycle is a remarkable process that occurs in women of reproductive age, typically lasting around 28 days. It involves a complex interplay of hormones, which regulate the growth and release of an egg from the ovaries and prepare the uterus for potential pregnancy.

The menstrual cycle consists of four main phases:

1. **Menstruation:** The cycle begins with menstruation, characterized by the shedding of the uterine lining. This phase usually lasts around 3 to 7 days and is accompanied by varying degrees of discomfort or cramping for some women.
2. **Funicular Phase:** Following menstruation, the funicular phase begins. During this phase, the pituitary gland releases follicle-stimulating hormone (FSH), which stimulates the development of follicles in the ovaries. One follicle will eventually mature and release an egg.
3. **Ovulation:** Midway through the menstrual cycle, ovulation occurs. A surge of luteinizing hormone (LH) triggers the release of the mature egg from the ovary. This is the most

fertile phase of the cycle, and conception is possible during this time.

4. **Luteal Phase:** After ovulation, the luteal phase begins. The ruptured follicle transforms into a structure called the corpus luteum, which produces progesterone to prepare the uterus for potential pregnancy. If fertilization doesn't occur, hormone levels drop, and the uterine lining begins to shed, initiating a new menstrual cycle.

Common Hormonal Imbalances in Women

Hormonal imbalances can occur due to various factors, including stress, diet, lifestyle choices, and underlying health conditions. These imbalances can lead to a range of symptoms and health issues that impact a woman's quality of life. Let's explore some common hormonal imbalances that women may experience:

1. **Estrogen Dominance:** Estrogen dominance occurs when there is an excess of estrogen relative to progesterone in the body. This imbalance can lead to symptoms such as heavy or irregular periods, mood swings, breast tenderness, and weight gain.
2. **Polycystic Ovary Syndrome (PCOS):** PCOS is a hormonal disorder characterized by imbalances in sex hormones, particularly elevated levels of androgens (male hormones). Women with PCOS may experience irregular periods, ovarian cysts, acne, excessive hair growth, and fertility issues.
3. **Hypothyroidism:** Hypothyroidism occurs when the thyroid gland doesn't produce enough thyroid hormones. Common symptoms include fatigue, weight gain, hair loss, cold intolerance, and menstrual irregularities.
4. **Hyperthyroidism:** Hyperthyroidism, on the other hand, involves an overactive thyroid gland that produces an excess of thyroid hormones. Symptoms may include weight loss, rapid heartbeat, anxiety, heat intolerance, and irregular menstrual cycles.

5. **Adrenal Imbalances:** Chronic stress can lead to imbalances in adrenal hormones such as cortisol and DHEA. Adrenal imbalances can cause fatigue, mood swings, sleep disturbances, and a disrupted menstrual cycle.

Natural Approaches to Balancing Hormones

Fortunately, several natural approaches can help restore hormonal balance and alleviate symptoms associated with hormonal imbalances. Here are some strategies to consider:

1. **Healthy Diet:** Opt for a balanced diet rich in whole foods, including fruits, vegetables, lean proteins, and healthy fats. Reduce processed foods, refined sugars, and artificial additives, as they can contribute to hormonal disruptions.
2. **Stress Management:** Chronic stress can disrupt hormone production and balance. Incorporate stress-reducing practices such as meditation, deep breathing exercises, yoga, or engaging in activities you enjoy to support your overall well-being.
3. **Regular Exercise:** Engaging in regular physical activity has numerous benefits for hormonal health. It can help regulate insulin levels, reduce stress, promote better sleep, and support overall hormonal balance. Find activities that you enjoy and aim for at least 150 minutes of moderate-intensity exercise per week.
4. **Adequate Sleep:** Quality sleep is essential for hormonal balance. Aim for 7-8 hours of uninterrupted sleep each night to support healthy hormone production and regulation.
5. **Herbal Support:** Certain herbs have been traditionally used to support hormonal balance. Examples include chasteberry (Vitex agnus-castus) for menstrual irregularities, black cohosh for menopausal symptoms, and dong quai for hormonal imbalances.
6. **Supplements:** Some supplements may help support hormonal balance. Consult with a healthcare professional to determine which supplements, such as omega-3 fatty acids, vitamin D, or

evening primrose oil, may be beneficial for your specific needs.

7. **Lifestyle Modifications:** Adopting healthy lifestyle habits can contribute to hormonal balance. Avoid excessive alcohol consumption and smoking, as they can disrupt hormone production. Maintain a healthy weight, as excess body fat can contribute to hormonal imbalances.

Remember, it's essential to consult with a healthcare professional before making significant changes to your diet, exercise routine, or starting any supplements. They can provide personalized guidance based on your individual needs and health status.

By implementing these natural approaches, you can support hormonal balance and improve your overall well-being. Taking a holistic approach to hormone health can have a positive impact on your menstrual cycle regularity, fertility, mood stability, and overall quality of life.

Hormonal health is integral to a woman's overall well-being. By understanding the phases of the menstrual cycle, recognizing common hormonal imbalances, and exploring natural approaches to balance hormones, you are equipped with valuable knowledge to support your hormonal health journey.

Remember, each woman's hormonal health is unique, and what works for one person may not work for another. Be patient with yourself, listen to your body, and seek professional guidance when needed. With a proactive approach and self-care practices, you can optimize your hormonal health and enjoy a vibrant and balanced life.

In the next chapter, we will delve into the realm of reproductive health, exploring fertility awareness, preconception care, and pregnancy health. Get ready to embark on an enlightening journey into the realm of women's reproductive well-being!

CHAPTER 3: REPRODUCTIVE HEALTH

Reproductive health plays a vital role in a woman's life, encompassing the various aspects of fertility, preconception care, and pregnancy. In this chapter, we will explore the key factors that contribute to reproductive health, discuss fertility awareness methods, delve into the importance of preconception care, and provide guidance for maintaining a healthy pregnancy.

Understanding Fertility Awareness

Fertility awareness is a valuable tool for understanding your menstrual cycle, identifying fertile days, and optimizing your chances of conception. By tracking changes in your body and observing specific fertility signs, you can gain insights into your fertility window. Let's explore some of the key methods used in fertility awareness:

1. **Basal Body Temperature (BBT) Charting:** Basal body temperature refers to your body's lowest resting temperature. By tracking your BBT daily, you can detect subtle temperature changes that indicate ovulation has occurred.
2. **Cervical Mucus Observation:** Changes in cervical mucus consistency throughout the menstrual cycle can provide clues about fertility. Observing the quality and quantity of cervical mucus can help you identify fertile and infertile phases.
3. **Ovulation Predictor Kits (OPKs):** These kits detect the surge in luteinizing hormone (LH) that occurs 24-48 hours before ovulation. By using OPKs, you can predict your most fertile days and plan intercourse accordingly.

4. **Menstrual Cycle Tracking Apps:** There are various smartphone apps available that allow you to track your menstrual cycle, record symptoms, and predict fertile windows based on the information provided. These apps can be useful for gaining insights into your cycle patterns and fertility.

Preconception Care: Nurturing the Path to Pregnancy

Preconception care involves taking proactive steps to optimize your health and prepare your body for a healthy pregnancy. By focusing on preconception health, you can enhance your fertility, reduce the risk of complications, and lay a strong foundation for the well-being of both you and your future baby. Here are some essential aspects of preconception care:

1. **Balanced Nutrition:** Adopt a well-rounded, nutrient-dense diet that includes a variety of fruits, vegetables, whole grains, lean proteins, and healthy fats. Ensure you're getting adequate amounts of key nutrients such as folic acid, iron, calcium, and omega-3 fatty acids.
2. **Supplementation:** Consider taking prenatal vitamins or supplements recommended by your healthcare provider. These can help fill any nutritional gaps and ensure you're meeting the specific nutrient needs during preconception and early pregnancy.
3. **Manage Chronic Conditions:** If you have any existing health conditions, work closely with your healthcare provider to manage and optimize their control before conceiving. Conditions such as diabetes, thyroid disorders, and hypertension can impact fertility and pregnancy outcomes.
4. **Achieve a Healthy Weight:** Attaining a healthy weight is crucial for fertility and a healthy pregnancy. Excess weight can disrupt hormone balance and ovulation, while being underweight may affect fertility and nutrient stores. Strive for a body mass index (BMI) within the healthy range.
5. **Address Lifestyle Factors:** Avoid smoking, excessive alcohol consumption, and illicit drugs, as they can significantly impact

fertility and increase the risk of pregnancy complications. Additionally, limit your caffeine intake and ensure you're engaging in regular physical activity.

Maintaining a Healthy Pregnancy

Once you conceive, maintaining a healthy pregnancy becomes a priority. Here are some key considerations and strategies for promoting a healthy pregnancy:

1. **Prenatal Care:** Schedule regular prenatal check-ups with a healthcare provider experienced in obstetrics. These visits are essential for monitoring your health, tracking the baby's development, and addressing any concerns or complications that may arise.
2. **Healthy Lifestyle Choices:** Continue following a balanced diet, focusing on nutrient-dense foods and avoiding potentially harmful substances. Stay physically active with exercises approved by your healthcare provider and ensure you get enough rest and sleep.
3. **Emotional Well-being:** Pregnancy can bring about a range of emotions. Take care of your mental and emotional well-being by seeking support from loved ones, joining prenatal support groups, practicing relaxation techniques, and seeking professional help if needed.
4. **Education and Preparedness:** Educate yourself about pregnancy, childbirth, and newborn care. Attend childbirth education classes, read books, and seek information from reliable sources. Being informed and prepared can alleviate anxiety and promote confidence during pregnancy and childbirth.
5. **Self-care and Stress Management:** Pregnancy can be physically and emotionally demanding. Prioritize self-care activities such as gentle exercises, prenatal yoga, massage, meditation, and engaging in activities that bring you joy. Manage stress through relaxation techniques and support from loved ones.

Remember, every pregnancy is unique, and it's essential to consult with your healthcare provider throughout the process. They can provide personalized guidance, address your specific needs, and monitor your health and the well-being of your baby.

Reproductive health is a multifaceted aspect of a woman's life. By understanding fertility awareness methods, practicing preconception care, and maintaining a healthy pregnancy, you are taking proactive steps to support your reproductive well-being.

Remember, fertility and pregnancy journeys can be complex, and it's normal to encounter challenges along the way. Seek support, be patient with yourself, and trust in the wisdom of your body. With proper care, knowledge, and support, you can enhance your reproductive health and pave the way for a joyful and fulfilling journey to motherhood.

In the next chapter, we will explore the unique challenges and considerations of women's sexual health. Join us as we delve into this important aspect of overall well-being!

CHAPTER 4: WOMEN'S SEXUAL HEALTH

Sexuality is an integral part of a woman's overall well-being and identity. Women's sexual health encompasses a wide range of factors, including sexual desire, pleasure, reproductive health, and emotional well-being. In this chapter, we will explore the various aspects of women's sexual health, address common concerns, and provide guidance for nurturing a healthy and fulfilling sexual life.

Understanding Female Sexual Anatomy

A fundamental aspect of women's sexual health is an understanding of female sexual anatomy. Familiarizing yourself with the structures involved in sexual pleasure and reproduction can contribute to a positive sexual experience. Let's explore the key components of female sexual anatomy:

1. **Clitoris:** The clitoris is a highly sensitive organ located at the top of the vulva. It contains thousands of nerve endings and is a primary source of sexual pleasure.
2. **Vagina:** The vagina is a muscular canal that connects the uterus to the external genitalia. It plays a crucial role in sexual intercourse and childbirth.
3. **G-Spot:** The G-spot is an area of heightened sensitivity located on the front wall of the vagina. Stimulating this area can lead to intense sexual pleasure and potentially result in female ejaculation.
4. **Ovaries:** The ovaries are responsible for producing eggs and releasing hormones, such as estrogen and progesterone.
5. **Uterus:** The uterus, also known as the womb, is a pear-shaped organ where a fertilized egg implants and develops during pregnancy.

Common Concerns and Conditions

Women may experience a variety of concerns and conditions related to their sexual health. Addressing these concerns can contribute to a more fulfilling and satisfying sexual life. Here are some common issues that women may encounter:

1. **Low Sexual Desire:** Decreased sexual desire can occur due to various factors, including hormonal changes, stress, relationship issues, or underlying medical conditions. Open communication with your partner and healthcare provider is crucial in addressing this concern.
2. **Painful Intercourse:** Pain during intercourse, known as dyspareunia, can have physical or psychological causes. Vaginal dryness, infections, pelvic floor muscle dysfunction, or emotional factors may contribute to this condition.
3. **Vaginal Dryness:** Vaginal dryness is often associated with hormonal changes, such as those experienced during menopause. It can cause discomfort and pain during sexual activity. Lubricants and hormonal therapies may help alleviate this symptom.
4. **Orgasmic Difficulties:** Difficulty reaching orgasm, known as anorgasmia, can result from physical, psychological, or relationship factors. Exploring different techniques, seeking therapy, or addressing underlying issues can help improve sexual satisfaction.
5. **Sexual Trauma and Emotional Wellness:** Past experiences of sexual trauma can impact a woman's sexual health and well-being. Seeking professional help and engaging in therapy can assist in healing and reclaiming a positive sexual identity.

Nurturing a Healthy and Fulfilling Sexual Life

Creating a healthy and fulfilling sexual life involves various factors, including communication, self-care, and intimacy. Here are some strategies to promote women's sexual health and well-being:

1. **Open Communication:** Establish open and honest communication with your partner regarding your desires, boundaries, and concerns. Effective communication can foster a deeper understanding and enhance sexual intimacy.
2. **Self-Exploration and Body Awareness:** Take time to explore your own body, desires, and preferences. Self-pleasure and self-exploration can increase body awareness, enhance sexual pleasure, and provide valuable information to share with your partner.
3. **Emotional Well-being:** Emotional well-being is vital for healthy sexual relationships. Addressing emotional concerns, seeking therapy if needed, and nurturing self-love and acceptance can positively impact sexual health.
4. **Sensate Focus:** Sensate focus exercises involve non-sexual touch and exploration of the body, allowing couples to focus on sensations and pleasure without the pressure of orgasm or performance. These exercises can enhance intimacy and strengthen emotional connections.
5. **Intimacy Beyond Intercourse:** Sexual intimacy extends beyond intercourse. Engage in various forms of intimacy, such as cuddling, kissing, sensual massages, or engaging in shared activities that bring you closer together.
6. **Seek Professional Help:** If concerns or conditions persist, consider seeking professional help from a healthcare provider or therapist specializing in sexual health. They can provide guidance, offer treatment options, and address any underlying medical or psychological issues.

Women's sexual health encompasses various dimensions that contribute to overall well-being, pleasure, and intimate connections. By understanding female sexual anatomy, addressing common concerns, and nurturing a healthy and fulfilling sexual life, you can cultivate a positive and empowering relationship with your sexuality.

Remember, every woman's journey is unique, and it's important to prioritize self-care, communication, and self-acceptance. Seek support when needed, embrace your desires and boundaries, and engage in open and honest conversations with your partner. Through this holistic approach, you can navigate the complexities of women's sexual health and create a fulfilling and satisfying sexual life.

In the next chapter, we will delve into the realm of mental health and explore strategies for maintaining emotional well-being. Join us as we discuss the significance of mental health and provide practical tips for self-care and resilience.

CHAPTER 5: MENTAL HEALTH AND WELL-BEING FOR WOMEN

Mental health is a crucial aspect of overall well-being, and it plays a significant role in women's lives. In this chapter, we will explore the unique challenges women may face in relation to mental health, discuss strategies for maintaining positive mental well-being, and provide guidance for coping with common mental health concerns.

Understanding Women's Mental Health

Women may experience distinct mental health challenges due to various factors, including hormonal fluctuations, societal expectations, reproductive events, and life transitions. It's essential to understand and address these challenges to promote mental well-being. Let's explore some key aspects of women's mental health:

1. **Hormonal Influences:** Hormonal changes throughout a woman's life, such as during puberty, menstrual cycles, pregnancy, and menopause, can impact mood, emotions, and overall mental well-being. Understanding these influences can help women navigate and manage their mental health effectively.

2. **Societal Pressures:** Women often face societal pressures related to body image, career expectations, caregiving responsibilities, and gender roles. These pressures can contribute to stress, anxiety, and feelings of inadequacy. Challenging and redefining societal norms can promote positive mental health.

3. **Reproductive Events:** Reproductive events like pregnancy, childbirth, and postpartum periods can bring about unique

mental health challenges. Conditions such as postpartum depression and anxiety may occur during this time. Early detection, support, and appropriate interventions are crucial for women's mental well-being.

Maintaining Positive Mental Well-being

Maintaining positive mental well-being is essential for women to thrive and lead fulfilling lives. Here are some strategies that can help promote positive mental health:

1. **Self-care:** Prioritize self-care activities that nourish your mind, body, and soul. Engage in activities you enjoy, practice relaxation techniques, establish healthy boundaries, and make time for hobbies, social connections, and self-reflection.
2. **Support Network:** Cultivate and nurture a support network of trusted friends, family members, or support groups. Having a safe space to share your thoughts, feelings, and experiences can provide validation, encouragement, and emotional support.
3. **Healthy Lifestyle:** Adopt a healthy lifestyle that includes regular physical exercise, a balanced diet, adequate sleep, and stress management techniques. Physical activity releases endorphins, improves mood, and reduces stress. A nutritious diet and sufficient sleep support overall well-being.
4. **Mindfulness and Relaxation:** Practice mindfulness techniques such as meditation, deep breathing exercises, or yoga to cultivate a sense of calm and reduce anxiety. These practices can help manage stress, increase self-awareness, and promote mental well-being.

Coping with Common Mental Health Concerns

Women may experience various mental health concerns throughout their lives. Here are some common mental health conditions and strategies for coping:

1. **Anxiety Disorders:** Anxiety disorders, including generalized anxiety disorder, panic disorder, and social anxiety disorder, are prevalent among women. Seek professional help, practice relaxation techniques, challenge negative thoughts, and consider therapy or medication if needed.
2. **Depression:** Depression affects women at a higher rate than men. Reach out for support, maintain a healthy routine, engage in activities that bring joy, and consider therapy or medication as appropriate. Don't hesitate to seek professional help when needed.
3. **Body Image Issues:** Many women struggle with body image issues, which can negatively impact mental health. Focus on self-acceptance, challenge societal beauty standards, surround yourself with positive influences, and seek professional help if body image concerns become overwhelming.
4. **Perinatal Mental Health:** Pregnancy and the postpartum period can bring about perinatal mental health concerns like postpartum depression and anxiety. Seek early screening, establish a support network, prioritize self-care, and consider therapy or medication if necessary.
5. **Trauma and PTSD:** Women may experience trauma and develop post-traumatic stress disorder (PTSD). Seek professional help, consider trauma-focused therapy, practice self-care, engage in grounding techniques, and connect with support groups for survivors of trauma.

Remember, mental health is a continuum, and everyone's experiences are unique. If you or someone you know is struggling with mental health concerns, reach out to healthcare professionals or mental health organizations for guidance, support, and appropriate interventions.

Maintaining positive mental health and well-being is crucial for women to lead fulfilling lives. By understanding the unique challenges women may face, implementing strategies for maintaining positive mental well-being, and seeking appropriate support, women can enhance their overall quality of life.

In the next chapter, we will explore strategies for promoting physical fitness and well-being. Join us as we discuss the importance of regular exercise, healthy lifestyle habits, and tips for incorporating fitness into your daily routine.

CHAPTER 6: PHYSICAL FITNESS AND WELL-BEING FOR WOMEN

Physical fitness is a vital component of overall well-being for women. Regular exercise, healthy lifestyle habits, and taking care of your body can contribute to improved physical health, mental well-being, and a higher quality of life. In this chapter, we will explore the importance of physical fitness for women, discuss different types of exercises, and provide tips for incorporating fitness into your daily routine.

The Importance of Physical Fitness for Women

Regular physical activity offers numerous benefits for women's health. Here are some key reasons why physical fitness is important:

1. **Cardiovascular Health:** Engaging in cardiovascular exercises, such as brisk walking, jogging, cycling, or swimming, can improve heart health, strengthen the cardiovascular system, and reduce the risk of heart disease.
2. **Weight Management:** Regular exercise, combined with a balanced diet, can help women maintain a healthy weight or achieve weight loss goals. Physical activity increases calorie expenditure, boosts metabolism, and builds lean muscle mass.
3. **Bone Health:** Weight-bearing exercises, like walking, dancing, or weightlifting, help strengthen bones and reduce the risk of osteoporosis and fractures, especially important for women as they age.
4. **Mental Well-being:** Physical activity releases endorphins, which promote feelings of happiness and reduce stress and

anxiety. Regular exercise can improve mood, enhance self-esteem, and contribute to better mental well-being.

5. **Hormonal Balance:** Physical fitness can help regulate hormonal balance in women, leading to improved menstrual health, reduced symptoms of premenstrual syndrome (PMS), and increased fertility.

Types of Exercises for Women

There are various types of exercises that women can incorporate into their fitness routine. It's important to choose activities that align with your interests, fitness level, and personal preferences. Here are some common types of exercises:

1. **Cardiovascular Exercises:** These exercises focus on elevating the heart rate and improving cardiovascular health. Examples include brisk walking, running, cycling, swimming, aerobic classes, and dancing.
2. **Strength Training:** Strength training exercises involve resistance training to build muscle strength and endurance. This can be done using free weights, weight machines, resistance bands, or bodyweight exercises like push-ups, squats, and lunges.
3. **Flexibility and Stretching:** Flexibility exercises help improve joint mobility, muscle flexibility, and overall range of motion. Activities like yoga, Pilates, and stretching exercises can enhance flexibility and promote relaxation.
4. **Balance and Stability Exercises:** These exercises aim to improve balance, coordination, and stability, reducing the risk of falls and injuries. Examples include yoga, tai chi, and specific balance exercises like standing on one leg or using balance boards.

Incorporating Fitness into Your Daily Routine

Finding time for physical fitness can be challenging, but small changes can make a significant difference. Here are some tips for incorporating fitness into your daily routine:

1. **Set Realistic Goals:** Define specific, measurable, achievable, relevant, and time-bound (SMART) fitness goals. Start with small milestones and gradually increase the intensity and duration of your workouts.
2. **Find Activities You Enjoy:** Choose activities that you genuinely enjoy and look forward to. It could be dancing, swimming, hiking, or joining a sports team. When you enjoy the exercise, it becomes easier to stay motivated.
3. **Make it a Habit:** Schedule regular exercise sessions in your weekly calendar and treat them as non-negotiable appointments with yourself. Consistency is key to reaping the benefits of physical fitness.
4. **Be Active Throughout the Day:** Look for opportunities to be active throughout the day, such as taking the stairs instead of the elevator, walking or cycling instead of driving short distances, or incorporating short bursts of exercise during work breaks.
5. **Seek Accountability and Support:** Find a workout buddy or join fitness classes or groups to stay motivated and accountable. Having someone to exercise with can make the experience more enjoyable and help you stay on track.
6. **Listen to Your Body:** Pay attention to your body's signals and adjust your exercise routine accordingly. Rest when needed, and consult a healthcare professional if you experience any pain or discomfort during exercise.

Physical fitness is essential for women's overall well-being. By incorporating regular exercise, choosing activities you enjoy, and making fitness a part of your daily routine, you can experience numerous physical and mental health benefits. Remember to start gradually, listen to your body, and seek professional guidance if needed.

In the next chapter, we will discuss nutrition and healthy eating habits for women. Join us as we explore the importance of a balanced diet, key nutrients for women's health, and strategies for making nutritious food choices.

CHAPTER 7: NUTRITION AND HEALTHY EATING HABITS FOR WOMEN

Proper nutrition is crucial for women's health and well-being. A balanced diet that includes essential nutrients supports overall physical health, mental well-being, and helps prevent chronic diseases. In this chapter, we will explore the importance of nutrition for women, discuss key nutrients, and provide tips for developing healthy eating habits.

The Importance of Nutrition for Women

Good nutrition plays a vital role in maintaining optimal health for women. Here are some key reasons why nutrition is important:

1. **Overall Health and Well-being:** Proper nutrition provides the necessary nutrients for the body to function optimally. It supports organ function, boosts the immune system, and contributes to overall well-being.
2. **Energy and Stamina:** A balanced diet provides the energy required for daily activities and helps maintain stamina throughout the day. Nutrient-dense foods fuel the body and promote vitality.
3. **Disease Prevention:** A healthy diet can help reduce the risk of chronic diseases such as heart disease, diabetes, certain types of cancer, and osteoporosis. Nutrient-rich foods contain antioxidants, phytochemicals, and other compounds that protect against cellular damage and inflammation.
4. **Hormonal Balance:** Adequate nutrition is essential for maintaining hormonal balance in women. Nutrients such as

omega-3 fatty acids, vitamins, and minerals play a role in regulating hormone production and function.

Key Nutrients for Women's Health

Women have specific nutrient requirements due to factors such as menstruation, pregnancy, lactation, and menopause. Here are some key nutrients that are particularly important for women:

1. **Calcium:** Calcium is essential for bone health and reducing the risk of osteoporosis. Good sources of calcium include dairy products, leafy greens, fortified plant-based milk, and calcium supplements if necessary.
2. **Iron:** Iron is necessary for the production of red blood cells and preventing iron deficiency anemia. Sources of iron include lean meats, poultry, fish, legumes, leafy greens, and fortified cereals.
3. **Folate:** Folate, or folic acid, is important for reproductive health, particularly during pregnancy, as it supports proper fetal development. Good sources of folate include leafy greens, citrus fruits, legumes, fortified grains, and prenatal supplements.
4. **Omega-3 Fatty Acids:** Omega-3 fatty acids, such as those found in fatty fish (e.g., salmon, mackerel, sardines), walnuts, flaxseeds, and chia seeds, have anti-inflammatory properties and support heart health, brain function, and hormonal balance.
5. **Vitamin D:** Vitamin D is necessary for bone health and immune function. Exposure to sunlight, fortified dairy products, fatty fish, and vitamin D supplements can help maintain adequate levels.

Developing Healthy Eating Habits

Developing healthy eating habits is key to maintaining proper nutrition. Here are some tips to help women develop a balanced and nourishing diet:

1. **Eat a Variety of Foods:** Include a wide range of fruits, vegetables, whole grains, lean proteins, and healthy fats in your diet. Aim for a colorful plate that represents different food groups.
2. **Portion Control:** Be mindful of portion sizes to maintain a healthy weight. Use smaller plates, measure servings, and pay attention to hunger and fullness cues.
3. **Hydration:** Drink an adequate amount of water throughout the day to stay hydrated. Limit sugary beverages and prioritize water as your main source of hydration.
4. **Limit Added Sugars and Processed Foods:** Minimize the consumption of foods high in added sugars, refined grains, and unhealthy fats. Opt for whole foods and prepare meals at home as much as possible.
5. **Meal Planning and Preparation:** Plan your meals and snacks ahead of time to ensure balanced nutrition and avoid impulsive food choices. Prep meals in advance and keep healthy snacks readily available.
6. **Mindful Eating:** Practice mindful eating by savoring each bite, paying attention to hunger and fullness cues, and avoiding distractions while eating. This helps foster a healthier relationship with food.
7. **Seek Professional Guidance:** If you have specific dietary concerns or health conditions, consider consulting a registered dietitian or healthcare professional who can provide personalized guidance and advice.

Nutrition plays a crucial role in women's health and well-being. By prioritizing a balanced diet that includes key nutrients, developing healthy eating habits, and being mindful of food choices, women can optimize their physical health, support hormonal balance, and reduce the risk of chronic diseases.

In the next chapter, we will delve into the topic of self-care and stress management for women. Join us as we explore strategies for promoting self-care, maintaining emotional well-being, and managing stress effectively.

CHAPTER 8: SELF-CARE AND STRESS MANAGEMENT FOR WOMEN

Self-care and stress management are essential components of maintaining overall well-being for women. In today's fast-paced world, it's crucial to prioritize self-care practices that promote physical, mental, and emotional health. In this chapter, we will explore the importance of self-care, discuss strategies for managing stress, and provide tips for incorporating self-care into your daily life.

The Importance of Self-Care for Women

Self-care refers to intentional actions and practices that prioritize your well-being and nurture your physical, mental, and emotional health. It involves recognizing your needs, setting boundaries, and engaging in activities that replenish and rejuvenate you. Here are some reasons why self-care is important for women:

1. **Stress Reduction:** Engaging in self-care activities can help reduce stress levels and promote relaxation. It allows you to recharge and replenish your energy, enabling you to better cope with daily challenges.

2. **Mental and Emotional Well-being:** Self-care practices contribute to improved mental and emotional health. They provide opportunities for self-reflection, self-compassion, and self-expression, fostering a positive mindset and emotional resilience.

3. **Enhanced Productivity and Focus:** Taking time for self-care can boost productivity and enhance focus. When you prioritize self-

care, you give yourself the necessary mental and physical breaks, which can improve concentration and performance in other areas of your life.

4. **Improved Relationships:** By taking care of your own well-being, you are better equipped to nurture and maintain healthy relationships. Self-care allows you to show up as your best self, fostering stronger connections with others.

Strategies for Managing Stress

Stress is a common experience for many women, and effective stress management is crucial for overall well-being. Here are some strategies to help manage and reduce stress:

1. **Identify Stress Triggers:** Recognize the situations, events, or people that tend to trigger stress for you. Awareness is the first step in effectively managing stress.

2. **Practice Relaxation Techniques:** Incorporate relaxation techniques into your routine, such as deep breathing exercises, meditation, progressive muscle relaxation, or engaging in activities that bring you joy and calmness.

3. **Time Management:** Prioritize tasks, set realistic goals, and learn to delegate when necessary. Effective time management can help reduce feelings of overwhelm and create a sense of control.

4. **Healthy Boundaries:** Establish and maintain healthy boundaries in your personal and professional life. Learn to say no when needed and prioritize your own needs and well-being.

5. **Physical Activity:** Engage in regular physical activity as a means of stress management. Exercise releases endorphins, reduces tension, and promotes overall well-being.

6. **Social Support:** Seek support from friends, family, or support groups. Sharing your feelings and experiences with others can provide emotional support and perspective.

Incorporating Self-Care into Your Daily Life

Self-care is not a luxury but a necessity. Here are some tips for incorporating self-care into your daily routine:

1. **Identify Your Needs:** Take time to identify your needs and preferences. What activities bring you joy, relaxation, or fulfillment? Make a list and incorporate them into your routine.

2. **Schedule Self-Care Time:** Dedicate specific time slots for self-care activities in your daily or weekly schedule. Treat them as non-negotiable appointments with yourself.

3. **Start Small:** Begin with small, manageable self-care activities. It could be as simple as taking a few minutes each day to practice deep breathing or enjoying a cup of herbal tea.

4. **Create a Self-Care Ritual:** Develop a self-care ritual that you can practice regularly, such as a morning meditation or an evening gratitude journaling session. Rituals help signal to your brain and body that it's time to relax and focus on self-care.

5. **Disconnect from Technology:** Set boundaries with technology and take regular breaks from screens. Disconnecting from digital devices can help reduce stress and promote mindfulness.

6. **Practice Self-Compassion:** Be kind to yourself and practice self-compassion. Treat yourself with the same care and compassion you would offer to a loved one.

Self-care and stress management are vital aspects of women's overall well-being. By prioritizing self-care, managing stress effectively, and incorporating self-care practices into your daily life, you can enhance your physical, mental, and emotional health. Remember, self-care is not selfish but necessary for you to show up as your best self and lead a fulfilling life.

In the next chapter, we will explore the topic of women's empowerment and self-confidence. Join us as we discuss strategies for building self-esteem, embracing your strengths, and cultivating a positive self-image.

CHAPTER 9: WOMEN'S EMPOWERMENT AND SELF-CONFIDENCE

Empowerment and self-confidence are essential for women to navigate through life with resilience, strength, and a sense of purpose. Embracing one's power and cultivating self-confidence can lead to personal growth, fulfillment, and the ability to overcome obstacles. In this chapter, we will explore the concept of women's empowerment, discuss strategies for building self-esteem, and provide tips for cultivating self-confidence.

Understanding Women's Empowerment

Women's empowerment involves recognizing and embracing one's innate power, rights, and abilities. It encompasses self-determination, autonomy, and the belief in one's worth and capabilities. Here are some key aspects of women's empowerment:

1. **Self-Awareness:** Women's empowerment begins with self-awareness. Understanding your values, strengths, and goals allows you to make conscious choices that align with your authentic self.

2. **Assertiveness:** Being assertive means expressing your thoughts, feelings, and needs with confidence and respect. It involves setting boundaries, advocating for yourself, and speaking up for what you believe in.

3. **Education and Knowledge:** Access to education and knowledge plays a crucial role in women's empowerment. It expands opportunities, enhances critical thinking, and equips women with the tools to make informed decisions.

4. **Supportive Networks:** Building and nurturing supportive networks is vital for women's empowerment. Surrounding yourself

with like-minded individuals who uplift and inspire you can provide encouragement and valuable resources.

Building Self-Esteem and Self-Worth

Self-esteem and self-worth are foundational to women's empowerment. Here are some strategies for building and nurturing self-esteem:

1. **Practice Self-Compassion:** Be kind to yourself and practice self-compassion. Treat yourself with understanding and acceptance, recognizing that nobody is perfect.
2. **Challenge Negative Self-Talk:** Become aware of negative self-talk and replace it with positive affirmations. Focus on your strengths, achievements, and unique qualities.
3. **Set Realistic Goals:** Set realistic and achievable goals that align with your values and passions. Celebrate small victories along the way to build confidence and self-belief.
4. **Embrace Failure as a Learning Opportunity:** See failure as a stepping stone to growth and learning. Embrace challenges, learn from setbacks, and use them as opportunities for personal development.

Cultivating Self-Confidence

Self-confidence is a key ingredient for women's empowerment. Here are some tips for cultivating self-confidence:

1. **Step Out of Your Comfort Zone:** Challenge yourself to step out of your comfort zone and embrace new experiences. Each time you take a risk, you expand your comfort zone and build confidence.
2. **Practice Self-Care:** Prioritize self-care practices that nurture your physical, mental, and emotional well-being. When you take care of yourself, you build a foundation of confidence and resilience.
3. **Celebrate Your Achievements:** Acknowledge and celebrate your accomplishments, no matter how small they may seem. Recognize your progress and give yourself credit for your efforts.

4. **Surround Yourself with Positive Influences:** Surround yourself with supportive and positive influences. Seek out mentors, role models, and friends who uplift and encourage you.

5. **Take Action Despite Fear:** Feel the fear and do it anyway. Taking action, even in the face of fear, builds confidence and shows you that you are capable of overcoming challenges.

6. **Practice Positive Body Image:** Embrace and celebrate your body as it is. Focus on what your body can do rather than how it looks, and engage in activities that promote body positivity and self-acceptance.

Women's empowerment and self-confidence are fundamental to leading a fulfilling and purposeful life. By embracing your power, building self-esteem, and cultivating self-confidence, you can navigate challenges with resilience, make choices that align with your authentic self, and inspire others around you.

In the next chapter, we will discuss the importance of maintaining healthy relationships and fostering a supportive community of women. Join us as we explore strategies for nurturing meaningful connections and creating a positive social network.

CHAPTER 10: MAINTAINING HEALTHY RELATIONSHIPS AND FOSTERING A SUPPORTIVE COMMUNITY OF WOMEN

Building and maintaining healthy relationships is crucial for women's well-being and personal growth. Surrounding yourself with a supportive community of women can provide emotional support, inspiration, and a sense of belonging. In this chapter, we will explore the importance of healthy relationships, discuss strategies for nurturing meaningful connections, and provide tips for fostering a supportive community of women.

The Importance of Healthy Relationships

Healthy relationships contribute to our overall happiness, emotional well-being, and personal development. Here are some reasons why healthy relationships are essential for women:

1. **Emotional Support:** Healthy relationships provide a safe space for emotional expression and support. They offer

comfort, empathy, and understanding during challenging
times.

2. **Self-Reflection and Growth:** Interacting with others in
healthy relationships helps us gain insight into ourselves.
Through meaningful connections, we receive feedback, learn
from different perspectives, and have opportunities for
personal growth.

3. **Inspiration and Motivation:** Healthy relationships can
inspire and motivate us to pursue our goals and dreams.
Seeing others thrive and succeed can ignite our own ambition
and drive.

4. **Accountability and Encouragement:** When we have healthy
relationships, we are surrounded by people who hold us
accountable and encourage us to be our best selves. They
support our endeavors and help us stay on track.

Strategies for Nurturing Healthy Relationships

Nurturing healthy relationships requires effort and intention. Here
are some strategies to help you foster and maintain meaningful
connections:

1. **Effective Communication:** Communication is the foundation
of any healthy relationship. Practice active listening, express
yourself honestly and respectfully, and be open to feedback.

2. **Mutual Respect:** Treat others with respect and expect the
same in return. Recognize and appreciate each other's
boundaries, values, and individuality.

3. **Empathy and Understanding:** Seek to understand others'
perspectives and experiences. Show empathy by validating
their feelings and demonstrating compassion.

4. **Quality Time:** Make time for meaningful connections.
Schedule regular get-togethers, engage in activities together,
and create shared experiences.

5. **Conflict Resolution:** Disagreements and conflicts are
inevitable in any relationship. Learn healthy ways to address

conflicts, practice compromise, and seek resolutions that benefit both parties.
6. **Support Each Other's Goals:** Encourage and support the aspirations and goals of the people in your life. Celebrate their achievements and provide encouragement during challenging times.

Fostering a Supportive Community of Women

In addition to individual relationships, fostering a supportive community of women can have a transformative impact. Here are some tips for creating and nurturing such a community:

1. **Seek Like-Minded Individuals:** Look for groups, organizations, or communities that align with your interests, values, or goals. Surrounding yourself with like-minded individuals creates a sense of belonging and camaraderie.
2. **Collaboration Over Competition:** Foster a culture of collaboration rather than competition within your community. Encourage uplifting and supportive interactions where women can celebrate each other's successes.
3. **Share Knowledge and Resources:** Offer your knowledge, skills, and resources to others in your community. Share insights, tips, and resources that can benefit and empower fellow women.
4. **Mentorship and Mentoring:** Seek out mentorship from experienced women who can guide and inspire you. Likewise, offer mentorship to younger or less experienced women, sharing your wisdom and supporting their growth.
5. **Engage in Supportive Activities:** Participate in activities and initiatives that promote support, empowerment, and personal development within your community. This can include workshops, conferences, or networking events.
6. **Embrace Diversity and Inclusion:** Create an inclusive and diverse community that welcomes women from different backgrounds, experiences, and perspectives. Embrace and celebrate the richness that diversity brings.

Maintaining healthy relationships and fostering a supportive community of women are vital for personal growth, well-being, and empowerment. By nurturing meaningful connections, practicing effective communication, and embracing a collaborative spirit, you can build a network of support that empowers and uplifts you.

In the next chapter, we will conclude our journey by reflecting on the key takeaways and encouraging you to continue your pursuit of women's health, empowerment, and personal development.

CHAPTER 11: INTEGRATIVE AND COMPLEMENTARY THERAPIES

Integrative and complementary therapies (ICTs) are a broad range of health care approaches that are not part of conventional medicine. They are often used alongside conventional treatments, or in place of them, to help people manage their health and well-being.

ICTs can include a wide variety of practices, such as acupuncture, massage therapy, herbal medicine, and yoga. They are based on different theories and philosophies, and they can be used to treat a wide range of conditions.

Some ICTs have been shown to be effective in treating certain conditions, while others have not been studied as extensively. It is important to talk to your doctor before starting any ICT, to make sure that it is safe for you and that it will not interfere with any other treatments you are taking.

Here is a more detailed overview of some of the most common ICTs:

Acupuncture

Acupuncture is a traditional Chinese medicine (TCM) practice that involves inserting thin needles into specific points on the body. It is thought to work by stimulating the body's natural healing abilities. Acupuncture has been shown to be effective in treating a variety of conditions, including pain, nausea, and anxiety.

Massage therapy

Massage therapy is a hands-on therapy that involves applying pressure to the muscles and soft tissues of the body. It is thought to work by improving circulation, reducing pain, and promoting relaxation. Massage therapy has been shown to be effective in treating a variety of conditions, including pain, stress, and anxiety.

Herbal medicine

Herbal medicine is the use of plants to treat health conditions. There are thousands of different herbs that have been used for medicinal purposes for centuries. Some herbs have been shown to be effective in treating certain conditions, while others have not been studied as extensively. It is important to talk to your doctor before taking any herbal supplements, to make sure that they are safe for you and that they will not interfere with any other treatments you are taking.

Yoga

Yoga is a mind-body practice that combines physical postures, breathing exercises, and meditation. It is thought to work by improving flexibility, strength, and balance, as well as reducing stress and anxiety. Yoga has been shown to be effective in treating a variety of conditions, including pain, stress, and anxiety.

Other ICTs

There are many other ICTs that are not as well-known as the ones listed above. Some of these include:

Homeopathy

Naturopathy

Reiki

Traditional Chinese medicine

It is important to do your research before starting any ICT, to make sure that it is safe for you and that it will not interfere with any other treatments you are taking.

If you are interested in trying an ICT, it is important to find a qualified practitioner. There are many different organizations that can help you find a qualified practitioner, such as the National Center for Complementary and Integrative Health (NCCIH) and the American Association of Naturopathic Physicians (AANP).

It is also important to talk to your doctor before starting any ICT, to make sure that it is safe for you and that it will not interfere with any other treatments you are taking.

ICTs can be a helpful addition to conventional medicine. They can help people manage their health and well-being, and they can also help people cope with the side effects of conventional treatments. If you are interested in trying an ICT, it is important to do your research and to talk to your doctor first.

CHAPTER 12.
EMPOWERMENT AND SELF-ADVOCACY

Empowerment and self-advocacy are two important concepts that can help people improve their lives. Empowerment is the process of gaining control over one's life, while self-advocacy is the act of speaking up for one's own needs and interests.

Empowerment can be achieved through a variety of means, such as education, training, and support groups. It can also be achieved through personal development, such as learning to set goals and to make decisions. When people are empowered, they are better able to take control of their lives and to make positive changes.

Self-advocacy is an important skill for everyone to have. It allows people to speak up for their needs and interests, even when they are faced with challenges. Self-advocacy can be used in a variety of settings, such as at school, at work, and in the community.

There are many benefits to empowerment and self-advocacy. These include:

Increased self-esteem and confidence

Improved ability to make decisions

Increased control over one's life

Reduced stress and anxiety

Improved relationships with others

Increased opportunities for success

If you are interested in learning more about empowerment and self-advocacy, there are many resources available. You can find books, articles, and websites that provide information and tips on how to empower yourself and to advocate for your own needs. You can also find support groups and other organizations that can help you on your journey to empowerment.

Here are some specific steps you can take to empower yourself and to advocate for your own needs:

Learn about your rights. It is important to know what your rights are as a citizen, as a student, as an employee, and as a member of your community. This knowledge will help you to advocate for yourself when necessary.

Set goals. Once you know what your rights are, you can start to set goals for yourself. What do you want to achieve in your life? What changes do you want to make? Having goals will give you something to work towards and will help you to stay motivated.

Make decisions. Empowerment means taking control of your life. This means making decisions for yourself, even when they are difficult. Don't be afraid to make mistakes. Everyone makes mistakes, but it is important to learn from them.

Take action. Once you have set goals and made decisions, it is time to take action. This may mean talking to people, writing letters, or even protesting. Don't be afraid to speak up for yourself and for what you believe in.

Empowerment and self-advocacy are important skills that can help you improve your life. By learning about your rights, setting goals, making decisions, and taking action, you can become more empowered and more in control of your life.

Here are some additional tips for empowering yourself and advocating for your own needs:

Build a support network. Having people who support you can make a big difference in your ability to empower yourself and to advocate for your own needs. Find people who believe in you and who will help you to achieve your goals.

Don't be afraid to ask for help. If you are struggling to empower yourself or to advocate for your own needs, don't be afraid to ask for help. There are many people who are willing to help you, including friends, family, professionals, and support groups.

Don't give up. Empowerment and self-advocacy are not always easy. There will be times when you feel discouraged or frustrated. But it is important to remember that you are not alone and that you can achieve your goals if you don't give up.

CONCLUSION

Women's health is a broad topic that encompasses many different aspects of a woman's physical and mental well-being. It is important for women to be aware of their health and to take steps to maintain it.

There are many things that women can do to improve their health, including:

Eating a healthy diet

Exercising regularly

Getting enough sleep

Managing stress

Seeing a doctor for regular checkups

Women should also be aware of the specific health risks that they face, such as breast cancer, ovarian cancer, and heart disease. By taking steps to reduce their risk factors and to get regular screenings, women can help to protect their health.

There are many resources available to help women learn more about their health. These include books, websites, and organizations that provide information and support. Women should not hesitate to reach out for help if they have any questions or concerns about their health.

By taking care of their health, women can live long, healthy lives.

Here are some additional tips for women's health

Talk to your doctor about your family history. This can help your doctor identify any health risks that you may be at risk for.

Get regular checkups. This includes Pap tests, mammograms, and other screenings that are important for women's health.

Know your body. Pay attention to any changes in your health, such as changes in your menstrual cycle or changes in your breasts.

Take care of your mental health. Stress, anxiety, and depression can all affect a woman's physical health. Make sure to take care of your mental health by getting enough sleep, exercising, and talking to a therapist if you need to.

Be an advocate for yourself. Don't be afraid to ask questions of your doctor or to speak up for your needs. You are your own best advocate when it comes to your health.

By following these tips, women can take control of their health and live long, healthy lives.